Pregnant & Not Posing

A (Mostly) Serious Guide to Yoga for Mamas

Helen Talbott

Copyright © 2024, Helen Talbott

Disclaimer

The information contained in this book is for informational purposes only and is not intended to be a substitute for professional medical advice, diagnosis, or treatment. Always consult with your healthcare provider before starting any new exercise program, especially during pregnancy or postpartum. The author and publisher of this book disclaim any liability for any adverse effects arising from the use of the information contained herein.

Medical Disclaimer

This book does not provide medical advice and is not intended to be a substitute for professional medical care. Always consult with your healthcare provider before starting any new exercise program, especially during pregnancy or postpartum. You should not rely on this book for any medical diagnosis or treatment.

Limitation of Liability

The author and publisher of this book disclaim any liability for any damages or injuries arising from the use of the information contained herein. The information provided in this book is based on the author's experience and research, but it is not guaranteed to be accurate or complete. The author and publisher make no warranties, express or implied, regarding the accuracy, completeness, or safety of the information contained herein.

Changes to This Page

The author and publisher reserve the right to make changes to this page at any time.

Table of contents

Introduction

Why "Namaste, New Mama" Shouldn't Be Your Only Mantra (But It Can Help!)

Ditching the Downward-Facing Doula: How Yoga Fits into Your Birth Prep Plan (Without Breaking the Bank)

My Body is Changing, So Should My Yoga: Modifications for Every Trimester

From Warrior Goddess to Warrior Mama: Building Physical and Mental Strength

First Trimester Flow: Finding Grounding and Stability

Second Trimester Stretch: Opening Hips and Embracing Flexibility

Third Trimester Twists: Preparing for Birth with Relaxation and Ease

Bonus Ball: Poses for Common Pregnancy Discomforts (Morning Sickness, Back Pain, & More!)

Pranayama Power: Breathing Techniques for Every Trimester and Labor Stage

Downward-Facing Diapers: Recovering Gracefully with Postpartum Yoga (Because #NewMomLife is Real)

Rebuilding Your Core: Gentle Strength Training for New Mamas (Because Your Core is More Than Just Abs)

Mama & Mini Flow: Bonding with Baby Through Yoga Practices (Because Cuddles & Playtime Can Be Yoga Too!)

You Did It, Mama! Celebrating Your Journey and Looking Ahead

Appendix

Sample Yoga Routines for Each Trimester

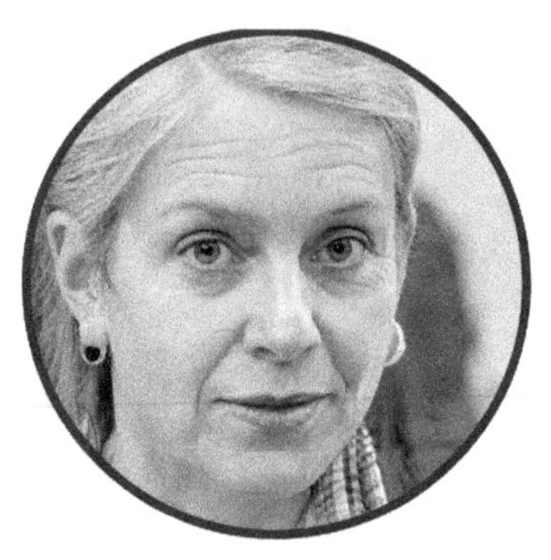

Hello there! I'm Helen Talbott, the author behind "Pregnant & Not Posing: A (Mostly) Serious Guide to Yoga for Mamas." As a dedicated yogi, I embarked on a journey to merge my passion for yoga with the transformative experience of pregnancy. With a mix of humor, practical advice, and a whole lot of love, I've crafted this guide to help fellow mamas navigate the beautiful, yet sometimes challenging, journey of pregnancy through the lens of yoga.

Drawing from my own experiences and insights gained from years of practicing yoga,

I aim to provide a holistic approach to pregnancy that goes beyond just physical poses. From soothing breathing exercises to gentle stretches tailored for each trimester, this book is designed to empower mamas-to-be to connect with their bodies, calm their minds, and embrace the incredible changes happening within.

But let's be real – pregnancy isn't always glamorous. That's why I've infused this guide with a healthy dose of humor and real-talk. Because whether you're dealing with morning sickness, swollen ankles, or just feeling like a beached whale, it's important to approach it all with a sense of humor and perspective.

So, to all the mamas out there – whether you're a seasoned yogi or a total newbie – I invite you to join me on this journey. Let's laugh, let's breathe, and let's embrace the beautiful chaos of pregnancy together. Namaste, mamas!

Introduction

Forget picture-perfect poses and impossible flexibility - motherhood is about real moments, real bodies, and a whole lot of laughter (along with some tears, let's be honest). This book isn't about nailing the "Insta-worthy" yoga mama image; it's about embracing the messy, beautiful journey of pregnancy with mindful movement and practical guidance.

So, put down the prenatal Instagram envy and grab your stretchy pants (comfy leggings work too) - we're diving into the world of yoga for mamas, the "mostly serious" kind. We'll explore poses that fit your changing body, breathing techniques to tame pregnancy anxieties, and practices that empower you for birth and beyond.

This book is your companion through every trimester, whether you're a seasoned yogi or just starting your practice. We'll chat about:

- **Why yoga rocks for pregnant mamas (even if you can't touch your toes)**
- **Adapting poses to accommodate your growing bump and unique needs**
- **Building strength and flexibility for a smoother birth experience**
- **Calming your mind and finding inner peace amidst the pregnancy roller coaster**
- **Recovering gracefully and bonding with your baby after delivery**

Chapter 1

Why "Namaste, New Mama" Shouldn't Be Your Only Mantra (But It Can Help!)

Picture this: You're scrolling through social media, bombarded by images of glowing pregnant women effortlessly holding perfect yoga poses, captions screaming "namaste, new mama!" and "find your inner zen!" While you may aspire to that level of serenity, let's be honest, reality feels more like "nausea, new mama!" and "find my inner strength to get out of bed!"

Fear not, fellow warriors-in-the-making! This book isn't here to shame you for not achieving picture-perfect prenatal bliss. Instead, we're here to celebrate the real, messy, and often hilarious journey of pregnancy with a healthy dose of yoga – **the "mostly serious" kind.**

So, let's ditch the unrealistic expectations and dive into the **why** behind prenatal yoga, embracing its benefits without the pressure of forced zen:

1. It's a Pregnancy Powerhouse: Yoga strengthens your core and pelvic floor, preparing them for the demands of birth. Think of it as building a badass internal scaffolding for your little one's arrival.

2. Flexibility Friend: As your bump grows, so does the need for some serious stretching. Yoga helps keep your muscles limber, reducing aches and pains and making everyday movements (like reaching for that dropped pacifier) a breeze.

3. Bye-Bye Back Pain: Hello, peaceful nights! Pregnancy often comes with lower back woes. Yoga postures, like cat-cow and child's pose, can ease discomfort and promote better sleep (because sleep is a luxury, mamas!).

4. Stress Slayer: Pregnancy is a whirlwind of emotions. Yoga, with its focus on breathwork and mindfulness, helps you manage anxiety, find inner peace, and even prepare for the mental challenges of labor.

5. Building Your Mama Village: Prenatal yoga classes can be a fantastic way to connect with other expecting mamas, creating a supportive community to share experiences, anxieties, and maybe even a few laughs (because laughter is the best medicine, especially when you're about to pee your pants from laughing).

Now, about that "namaste, new mama." While it might not be your sole mantra, there's power in acknowledging the calmness and strength within you. So, go ahead, say it with a wink, knowing that behind the "namaste" lies a fierce mama ready to rock this pregnancy journey, yoga mat (and maybe a few pickles) in hand.

Remember, this is your journey, your yoga, and your mantra. Let's embrace the real, the messy, and the beautifully imperfect together. Now, let's bend, breathe, and maybe even giggle our way into a more empowered pregnancy!

Chapter 2

Ditching the Downward-Facing Doula: How Yoga Fits into Your Birth Prep Plan (Without Breaking the Bank)

So, you're pregnant, excited, and maybe a little overwhelmed by the birth prep vortex. Birthing classes, doulas, hypnobirthing... it all sounds amazing, but your wallet is starting to sing the high notes of panic. Fear not, mama-to-be! Before you break the bank on a "Downward-Facing Doula," let's talk about how yoga can become your affordable and empowering birth preparation bestie.

Building Strength, Naturally:

Forget expensive gym memberships. Gentle yoga poses targeted at your core and pelvic floor muscles can create a foundation of strength for birth. Think of it as building your own internal power suit, minus the shoulder pads and uncomfortable Spanx.

Flexibility for the Win: As your bump grows, so does your need for some serious stretching. Yoga helps keep your muscles limber, reducing aches and pains and making everyday movements (like reaching for that dropped baby wipe) a breeze. Who needs expensive massage therapists when you can become your own contortionist (well, almost)?

Breathing Like a Boss: Let's talk about the real elephant in the room: labor contractions. While they might sound like your worst nightmare, mastering your breath can transform them into manageable waves. Yoga's focus on conscious breathing techniques like Ujjayi and Nadi Shodhana can equip you with the tools to navigate those contractions like a boss (while maybe channeling your inner Beyoncé in the process).

Mind Over Matter: Pregnancy emotions are a rollercoaster. Anxiety, stress, and fear can hijack your birth experience. Yoga, with its emphasis on mindfulness and meditation, helps you manage these emotions, find inner peace, and even build mental resilience for the challenges of labor. Think of it as building a mental shield against worry, all without shelling out for fancy meditation apps.

Community Connection: Feeling overwhelmed by the solo pregnancy journey? Prenatal yoga classes can be a fantastic way to connect with other expecting mamas, creating a supportive community to share experiences, anxieties, and maybe even a few laughs (because laughter is the best medicine, especially when you're about to pee your pants from laughing... again). It's like having built-in birth buddies without the hefty doula price tag.

Remember: Yoga is not a magic bullet, but it's a powerful tool in your birth preparation arsenal. It's affordable, accessible, and can be easily adapted to your individual needs and preferences. So, ditch the perfectionist pressure, grab your yoga mat (or comfy blanket), and embrace the "mostly serious" approach to prenatal yoga. You might just discover a badass mama within, ready to rock this birth, downward-facing doula or not!

Chapter 3

My Body is Changing, So Should My Yoga: Modifications for Every Trimester

Remember that picture-perfect prenatal yogi you saw on Instagram, effortlessly holding a handstand while radiating inner light? Yeah, let's just say her reality (and yours) probably involves more heartburn and bathroom breaks than blissful serenity. The good news is, yoga for pregnancy isn't about chasing unattainable poses; it's about **honoring your changing body and adapting your practice to every trimester.**

First Trimester: Nausea, fatigue, and that ever-present "what just hit me?" feeling might not scream "yoga time," but gentle movement can actually ease these discomforts. Stick to **grounding poses** like mountain pose, cat-cow, and supported child's pose. Modify downward-facing dog by placing your hands on a wall or chair for extra support. Remember, listening to your body is key, so take breaks and rest whenever needed.

Second Trimester: Ah, the "golden trimester" often brings newfound energy. Now's the time to **explore poses that open your hips and improve flexibility.** Warrior poses, modified triangle pose, and gentle hip circles can become your new best friends. Remember, as your belly grows, adjust poses by using blocks or bolsters for support and prioritize modifications that feel comfortable and safe.

Third Trimester: The home stretch can be demanding, with increased weight and fatigue. Don't be afraid to **downsize your practice and focus on relaxation and breathing techniques.** Supported reclined poses, child's pose variations, and gentle leg stretches can ease aches and pains. Pranayama techniques like Ujjayi and Nadi Shodhana can become your go-to tools for managing anxiety and preparing for labor.

Remember: Modifying isn't a sign of weakness; it's a sign of wisdom! Here are some general tips for every trimester:

- **Listen to your body:** If something feels uncomfortable, stop! Modify or rest as needed.
- **Use props:** Blocks, bolsters, blankets – they're your best friends! Use them for support, elevation, or even just padding those sensitive areas.
- **Hydrate:** Drink plenty of water before, during, and after your practice.
- **Breathe:** Focus on your breath throughout your practice. It's your anchor to calmness and can even help manage labor contractions.
- **Don't push yourself:** This isn't the time to break any personal records. Enjoy gentle movement and celebrate your body's incredible journey.

Remember, the goal isn't to impress anyone with your flexibility (or contortions). Embrace the "mostly serious" approach to prenatal yoga, modify with confidence, and enjoy the empowering journey of connecting with your changing body and preparing for motherhood, one mindful breath at a time.

Chapter 4

From Warrior Goddess to Warrior Mama: Building Physical and Mental Strength

Forget dainty flower poses – pregnancy is about fierce mama energy! While you might not be slaying mythical beasts (yet), this chapter is about channeling your inner warrior, building both physical and mental strength for the epic journey of birth and motherhood.

Strength from Within:

Pregnancy isn't just about the bump. It's about preparing your entire body for the demands of delivery and caring for a tiny human. Yoga poses like lunges, modified warriors, and squats can **build core and pelvic floor strength**, creating a foundation for labor and postpartum recovery. Think of it as forging your internal armor – one downward-facing dog at a time!

Flexibility for the Win: As your bump blossoms, so does your need for some serious stretching. Yoga helps keep your muscles limber, reducing aches and pains and making everyday movements (like reaching for that dropped toy) a breeze. Imagine yourself not as a stiff tree, but as a graceful willow, bending with the wind (and those inevitable tantrums).

Breath: Your Secret Weapon: Let's talk contractions – they might sound like your worst nightmare, but mastering your breath can transform them into manageable waves. Yoga's focus on conscious breathing techniques like Ujjayi and Nadi Shodhana equips you with the tools to navigate those surges like a warrior queen, channeling every exhale into power and focus.

Mental Grit, Mama Style: Pregnancy hormones are a rollercoaster. Anxiety, stress, and fear can hijack your birth experience. Yoga, with its emphasis on mindfulness and meditation, helps you manage these emotions, find inner peace, and build **mental resilience** for the challenges of labor and motherhood. Think of it as building a mental shield against worry, empowering you to face each moment with grace and strength.

Fueling Your Journey: Remember, even warriors need sustenance! Nourish your body with healthy foods and hydrate like a desert camel. This provides the energy you need for your practice, supports fetal development, and keeps you feeling your best. Listen to your body's cravings (within reason, of course – that third slice of cake might not be calling your name).

Remember: You are a warrior mama in the making. Your yoga practice is a tool to connect with your strength, cultivate resilience, and prepare for the incredible journey ahead. Embrace the power within, celebrate your changing body, and remember, even the fiercest warriors take breaks when needed. So grab your yoga mat (or comfy blanket), channel your inner goddess, and roar your way into a strong and empowered pregnancy!

Bonus Tip: Visualize yourself conquering labor like a warrior queen, using your breath as your weapon and your strength as your shield. This positive visualization can boost your confidence and empower you to approach birth with a warrior's spirit.

Chapter 5

First Trimester Flow: Finding Grounding and Stability

Welcome, mamas-to-be, to the first trimester! This exciting (and sometimes nauseous) phase lays the foundation for your journey. While your body undergoes amazing transformations, you might be feeling more like a seasick sailor than a grounded yogi. Don't worry, this chapter will guide you through a gentle flow designed to find stability and comfort in the early stages of pregnancy.

Embracing the Changes:

The first trimester is all about **listening to your body**. Fatigue, nausea, and heightened emotions are your companions. Remember, there's no shame in modifying poses or taking frequent breaks. Your goal is to create a peaceful and nourishing practice, not impress anyone (especially not that Instagram yogi with the perfect bump!).

Grounding Poses for Inner Calm:

- **Mountain Pose (Tadasana):** Stand tall with feet hip-width apart, root your feet into the ground, and feel your connection to the earth. This simple pose centers your mind and grounds your energy.

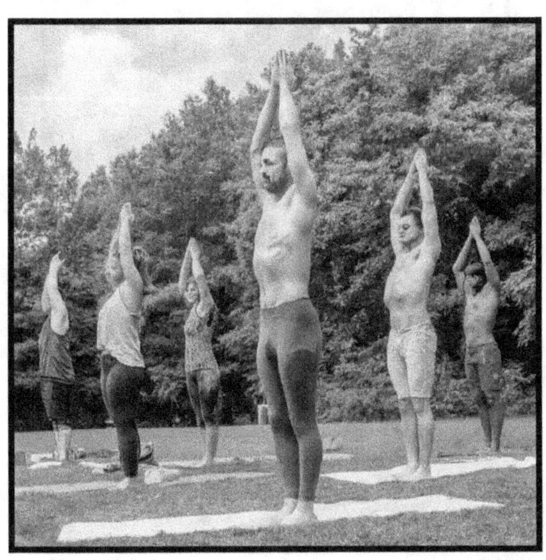

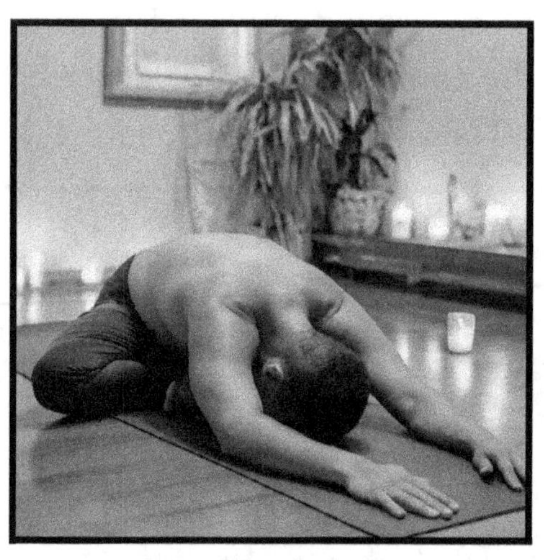

- **Supported Child's Pose (Balasana):** Kneel on the floor, sit back on your heels, and rest your forehead on the mat or a bolster. This relaxing pose eases nausea and fatigue, providing a safe haven for inward reflection.

- **Cat-Cow (Marjariasana-Bitilasana):** On all fours, arch your back as you inhale (cow) and round your spine as you exhale (cat). This gentle movement promotes spinal mobility and relieves backache.

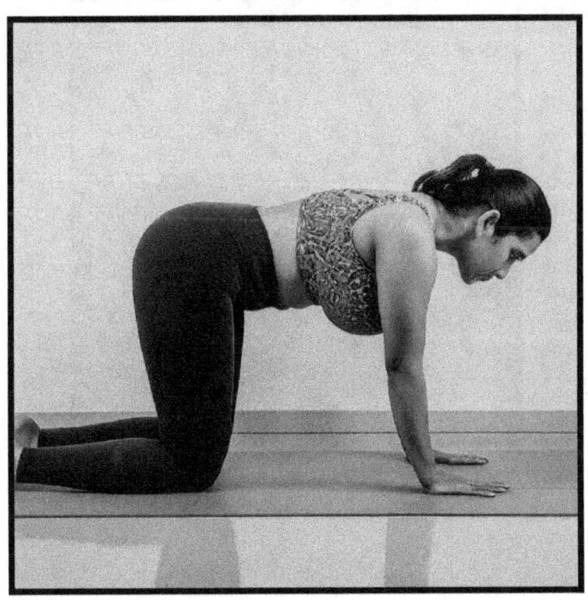

Gentle Stretches for Comfort:

- **Neck Rolls:** Slowly roll your head in a circular motion, releasing tension in your neck and shoulders.

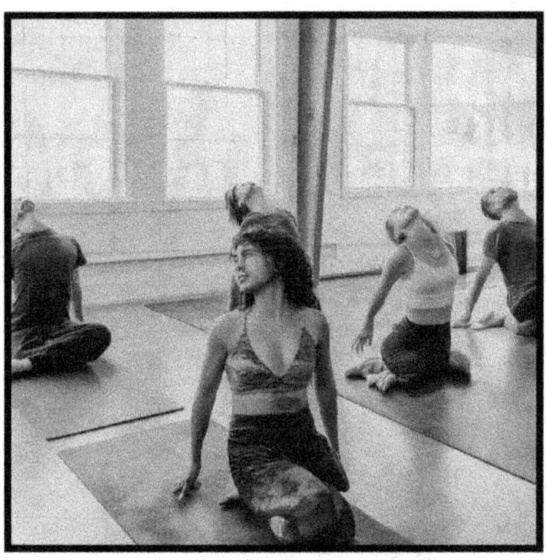

- **Wrist Circles:** Warm up your wrists with gentle forward and backward rotations.

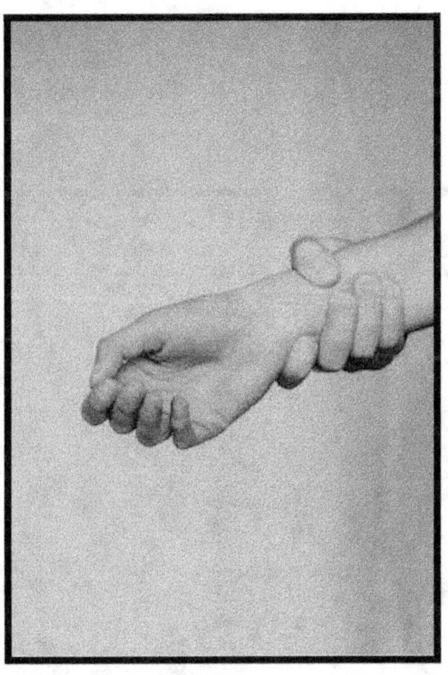

- **Modified Seated Forward Bends:** Sit on a chair or bolster, and slowly fold forward, lengthening your spine without straining. This stretch eases morning sickness and promotes relaxation.

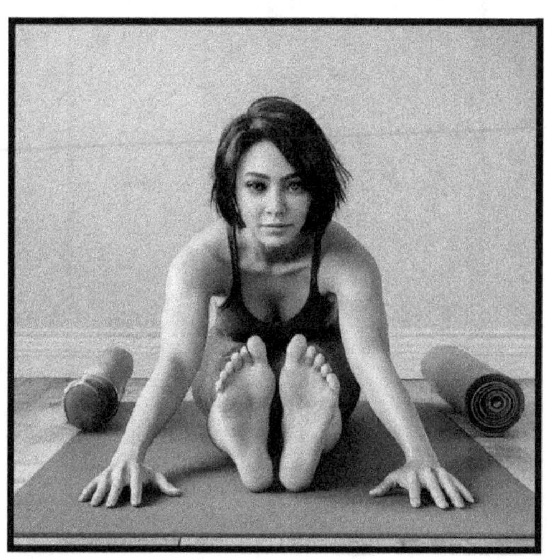

Pranayama for Peace:

- **Ujjayi Breath:** This ocean-like breath calms the mind and regulates your nervous system. Inhale and exhale through your nose with a slight constriction at the back of your throat.

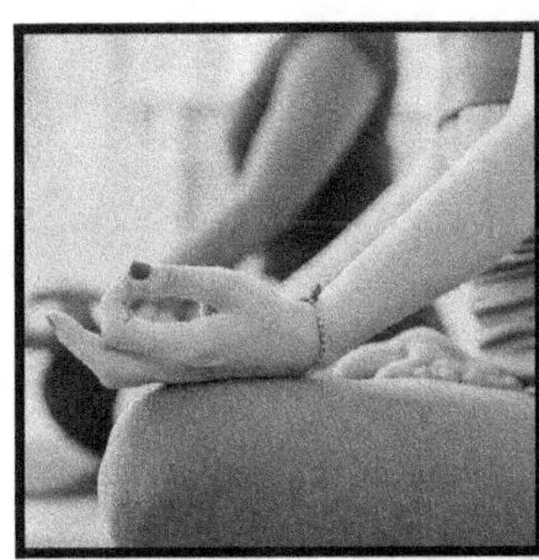 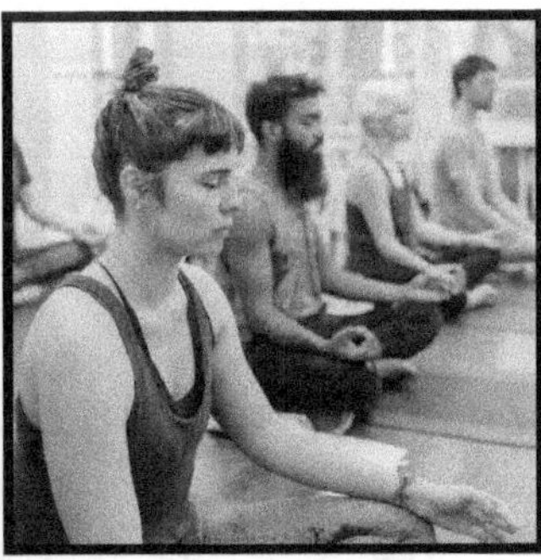

- **Alternate Nostril Breathing (Nadi Shodhana):** Close one nostril, inhale, close the other, exhale. Repeat on the other side. This calming breath balances your energy and promotes emotional stability.

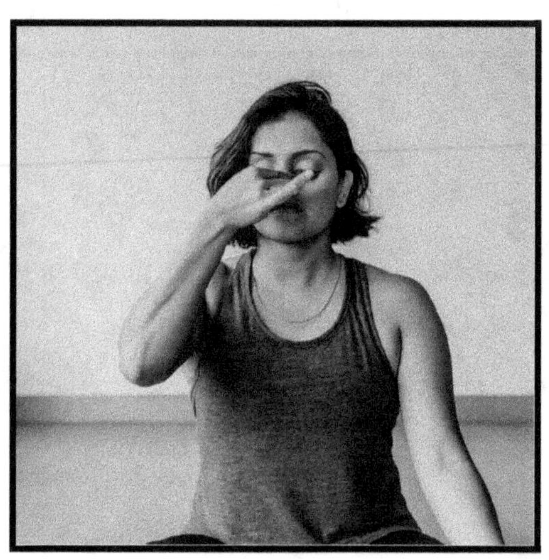

Remember:

- Listen to your body and modify poses as needed. Use props like bolsters, blankets, or blocks for support.
- Hydrate before, during, and after your practice.

- Breathe deeply and focus on the present moment.
- Be kind to yourself – this is a time for gentle movement and nurturing self-care.

This first trimester flow is just a starting point. Explore different poses, breathing techniques, and guided meditations that resonate with you. Remember, mama, this is your journey, so flow gracefully, find your inner stability, and enjoy the transformative power of yoga in the early stages of motherhood.

Chapter 6

Second Trimester Stretch: Opening Hips and Embracing Flexibility

Welcome, mamas-in-the-making, to the glorious (and sometimes glowy) second trimester! Your energy is returning, your bump is blossoming, and now's the perfect time to focus on **opening your hips and cultivating flexibility**. This chapter will guide you through a flow designed to prepare your body for the demands of labor while nurturing a sense of ease and joy in your practice.

Embracing the "Bump":

The second trimester brings exciting changes, including a growing belly and loosening joints. While this flexibility can benefit your practice, it's also important to maintain stability and listen to your body's limits. Remember, modifications are your best friends, so don't hesitate to adjust poses to accommodate your changing needs.

Opening Hips for Easier Delivery:

- **Malasana (Squat Pose):** Stand with feet hip-width apart, squat down as if sitting in an imaginary chair, keeping your back straight and toes turned slightly outward. This hip-opening pose prepares your pelvic floor for birth and strengthens your legs.

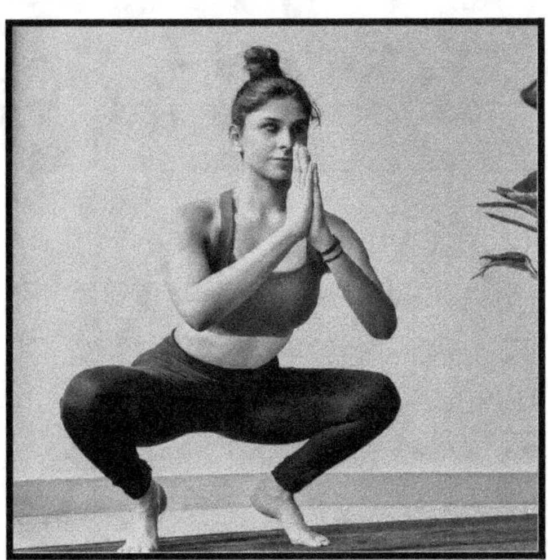

- **Butterfly Pose (Baddha Konasana):** Sit on the floor with soles of your feet together, knees bent and open wide. Gently press your knees down towards the floor, focusing on a deep hip stretch. This pose increases pelvic flexibility and reduces sciatica pain.

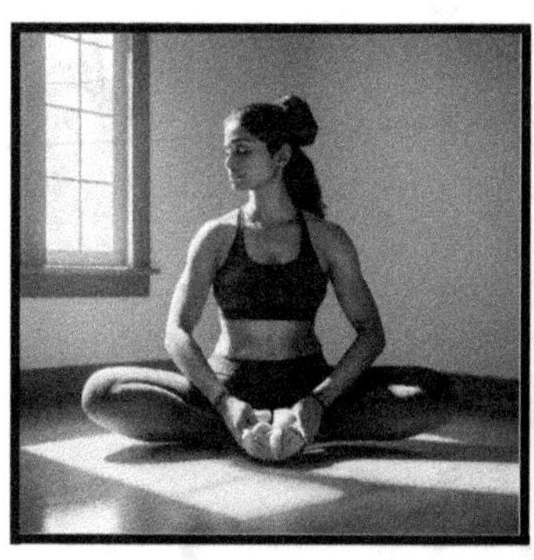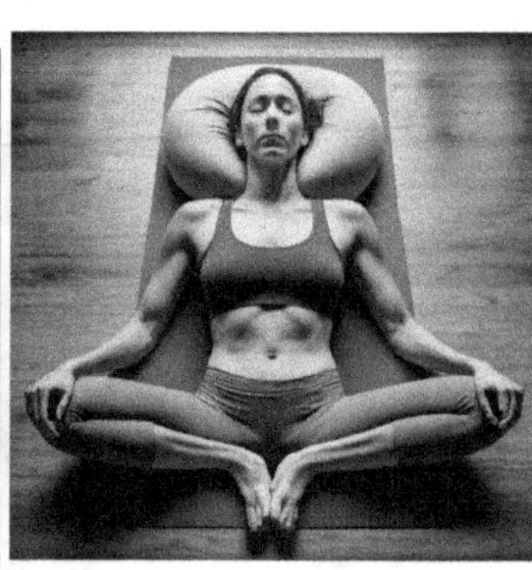

- **Figure-Four Stretch:** Lie on your back, bring one knee towards your chest, clasp your hands around your shin, and gently pull your thigh towards your body. Hold for a few breaths on each side, stretching your hip flexors and glutes.

Gentle Backbends for Relaxation:

- **Supported Bridge Pose (Setu Bandhasana):** Lie on your back with knees bent, feet flat on the floor. Lift your hips off the ground, supporting your lower back with a block or bolster. This gentle backbend opens your chest, alleviates fatigue, and improves posture.
- **Cat-Cow with Hip Circles:** On all fours, combine the familiar cat-cow movement with gentle hip circles. This combination promotes spinal mobility, releases tension, and increases hip flexibility.

Pranayama for Inner Balance:

- **Bhramari (Humming Bee Breath):** Close your ears and mouth, inhale deeply, and exhale slowly with a humming sound. This calming breath reduces anxiety, promotes relaxation, and soothes the mind.
- **Alternate Nostril Breathing (Nadi Shodhana):** As you did in the first trimester, close one nostril, inhale, close the other, exhale. Repeat on the other side.

This balancing breath harmonizes your energy and promotes emotional well-being.

Remember:

- Listen to your body and modify poses as needed. Use props to ensure proper alignment and comfort.
- Stay hydrated throughout your practice.
- Breathe deeply and focus on connecting with your body and your growing baby.
- Be patient and kind to yourself – flexibility takes time and practice.

This second trimester flow is an invitation to move with joy, open your hips for an easier delivery, and cultivate inner peace through mindful breathing. Embrace the changes, celebrate your blossoming body, and enjoy the transformative power of yoga on this wondrous journey of motherhood.

Chapter 7

Third Trimester Twists: Preparing for Birth with Relaxation and Ease

Welcome, mamas-in-full-bloom, to the glorious (and sometimes unwieldy) third trimester! Your bump is proudly prominent, your energy might be fluctuating, and birth feels closer than ever. This chapter guides you through a gentle flow designed to **prepare for birth with relaxation, ease, and a touch of playful twisting.**

Embracing Comfort and Modifications:

By now, your body whispers its limitations loud and clear. Honor them! Modify every pose, use plenty of props, and prioritize comfort over perfect alignment. This isn't about achieving peak yoga poses; it's about nurturing your well-being and preparing for birth with gentleness and acceptance.

Twists for Gentle Release:

- **Seated Spinal Twist (Ardha Matsyendrasana):** Sit on the floor with legs extended, bend one knee and bring the foot over the opposite thigh. Twist your upper body towards the bent knee, gazing over your shoulder. Repeat on the other side. This twist gently massages your spine and relieves back pain.

- **Supported Marjariasana (Cat Pose) with Twists:** On all fours, arch your back as you inhale (cow) and twist your upper body slightly to one side. Exhale as you round your spine and twist to the other side. Use a bolster for support under your knees or chest as needed. This dynamic stretch releases tension and improves spinal mobility.

- **Supported Reclined Figure-Four Twist:** Lie on your back with knees bent, bring one ankle over the opposite thigh. Gently twist your upper body towards the bent knee, gaze over your shoulder, and hold for a few breaths. Repeat on the other side. This relaxing twist opens your hips and soothes lower back discomfort.

Relaxation Poses for Inner Peace:

- **Supported Savasana (Corpse Pose):** Lie on your back with legs extended, arms at your sides, and palms facing upwards. Use bolsters or blankets to support your back, hips, and knees. Close your eyes and focus on your breath, allowing your body to completely surrender to relaxation. This is a restorative pose that calms the mind and eases pregnancy discomforts.
- **Supine Supported Child's Pose (Balasana):** Kneel on the floor, sit back on your heels, and rest your forehead on a bolster or stack of blankets. Relax your arms and shoulders, focusing on deep, peaceful breaths. This pose fosters inner peace and reduces anxiety.
- **Guided Meditation:** Find a quiet space and settle into a comfortable position. Close your eyes and listen to a guided

meditation for pregnancy, visualizing a calm and empowered birth experience. This practice promotes emotional well-being and prepares you for the mental challenges of labor.

Pranayama for a Calm Delivery:

- **Ujjayi Breath:** This ocean-like breath remains your trusty companion throughout pregnancy. Practice it throughout your flow and during labor contractions to remain calm and focused.
- **Kapalbhati (Breath of Fire):** Inhale and exhale rapidly through your nose for several rounds. This energizing breath can be practiced in short bursts to manage fatigue and maintain alertness during labor.

Remember:

- Listen to your body and modify poses as needed. There's no shame in resting or taking breaks.

- Stay hydrated throughout your practice and throughout the day.
- Breathe deeply and focus on connecting with your breath and your baby.
- Trust your body's incredible ability to give birth. Yoga is a tool to prepare and nurture, not a guarantee of a perfect birth experience.

Embrace this gentle flow as a time for inner peace, mindful preparation, and playful exploration. Remember, mama, you are strong, capable, and ready to birth your little one with grace and serenity. Relax, twist, breathe, and enjoy the final stretch of your beautiful pregnancy journey.

Chapter 8

Bonus Ball: Poses for Common Pregnancy Discomforts (Morning Sickness, Back Pain, & More!)

Pregnancy is a magical time, but let's be honest, it can also come with its fair share of discomforts. From nausea to backaches, heartburn to insomnia, these little annoyances can throw even the most zen mama off balance. But fear not, mama-to-be! Yoga can be your secret weapon to combat these common pregnancy woes and bring back a touch of comfort and ease.

Battling the Blahs:

- **Nausea:** Ginger is your friend! Sip on ginger tea before your practice, and try poses like Supported Child's Pose or Seated Cat-Cow with deep, calming breaths. Avoid inversions and intense poses that might trigger nausea.

- **Fatigue:** Gentle movement can actually boost your energy! Modified Sun Salutations, Warrior I & II variations, and supported reclined twists can combat fatigue and leave you feeling refreshed.

Back in Business (Without the Ache):

- **Lower Back Pain:** Supported Bridge Pose with bolsters under your hips and knees, Cat-Cow variations with gentle spinal movements, and Seated Spinal Twists with modifications can all bring relief to a strained lower back.
- **Sciatica:** Listen to your body! Avoid poses that aggravate the pain, and focus on gentle hip stretches like Butterfly Pose, Figure-Four Stretch, and supported reclined poses with knees elevated.

Other Common Grumbles:

- **Heartburn:** Avoid poses that compress your abdomen, like deep forward bends. Stick to Supported Child's Pose, Seated Spinal Twists, and reclined supported poses to keep the fire in your belly at bay.
- **Insomnia:** Wind down your day with a calming evening yoga routine. Supported Savasana with guided meditation, gentle seated stretches, and deep, relaxing breaths can prepare your body and mind for a restful sleep.

Remember:

- Listen to your body and modify poses as needed. Don't force anything that causes discomfort.
- Use props like bolsters, blankets, and blocks for support and proper alignment.
- Stay hydrated before, during, and after your practice.
- Breathe deeply and focus on relaxation and inner peace.

Chapter 9

Ujjayi Ain't Easy: Mastering the Breathwork for a Calm Delivery (But It's Worth It!)

Okay, mamas, let's be real: mastering Ujjayi breath can feel like trying to wrangle a mischievous toddler. That hissing ocean sound may seem elusive, but trust me, this breathwork is your secret weapon for a calmer, more empowered birth experience. So, let's ditch the frustration and dive into the why and how of mastering Ujjayi for pregnancy (and beyond!).

Why Ujjayi is Your Birth BFF:

- **Calming Queen:** Anxiety and fear can hijack your birth experience. Ujjayi's soothing rhythm regulates your nervous system, keeping you feeling centered and grounded. Think of it as your built-in stress-buster.

- **Pain Management Powerhouse:** Contractions might sound scary, but with Ujjayi, you can transform them into manageable waves. Deep, focused breaths allow you to manage discomfort and find strength within each surge.

- **Pushing Partner:** When it's time to push, Ujjayi becomes your guide. Coordinating your breath with each push optimizes oxygen flow, increases efficiency, and even reduces tearing (bonus!).

Mastering the Ujjayi Art Form:

- **The Sound:** Imagine fogging up a mirror with your warm breath. That's the gentle ocean-like sound you're aiming for. Inhale and exhale through your nose, constricting slightly at the back of your throat. Don't worry, it'll feel weird at first, but practice makes progress!
- **Start Simple:** Begin with seated breathing exercises, focusing on the sound and rhythm. Gradually incorporate Ujjayi into gentle movement (think modified Surya Namaskar) to connect breath and body.

- **Practice Makes Perfect (ish):** Don't expect overnight mastery. Integrate short Ujjayi practices into your daily routine to build awareness and control. Meditation apps and online tutorials can also be helpful guides.

Remember:

- **No Pressure:** Ujjayi intensity varies for everyone. Find a comfortable level that allows you to breathe deeply and rhythmically.
- **It's a Journey:** Be patient and kind to yourself. Mastering Ujjayi takes time and practice, so celebrate each small victory.
- **Modifications Rule:** Listen to your body and modify if needed. Open your mouth to breathe if necessary, especially during labor.

Ujjayi might not be your favorite part of yoga, but trust me, mastering it can be incredibly empowering. So, take a deep breath, embrace the practice, and experience the transformative power of Ujjayi in preparing for a calmer, more confident birth. Remember, mama, you've got this!

Chapter 10

Pranayama Power: Breathing Techniques for Every Trimester and Labor Stage

Forget fancy gym memberships and expensive equipment, mama! Your breath is your most powerful tool throughout pregnancy and birth. In this chapter, we'll explore different pranayama techniques (fancy word for yogic breathing) tailored to each trimester and labor stage, empowering you to navigate this incredible journey with grace and ease.

First Trimester:

- **Nadi Shodhana (Alternate Nostril Breathing):** Calms anxiety and balances your energy. Close one nostril, inhale, close the other, exhale. Repeat on the other side. Practice this throughout your day for inner peace.

- **Bhramari (Humming Bee Breath):** Reduces stress and promotes relaxation. Close your ears and mouth, inhale deeply, and exhale with a humming sound. Practice this before bed for a peaceful night's sleep.

Second Trimester:

- **Ujjayi Breath:** Your constant companion throughout pregnancy. This rhythmic breath calms your nervous system, prepares for labor, and even aids digestion. Practice it during your yoga routine and throughout your day.
- **Kapalbhati (Breath of Fire):** Energizes your body and mind. Inhale and exhale rapidly through your nose for several rounds. Use this short burst of energy to combat fatigue or sluggishness.

Third Trimester:

- **Ujjayi Variations:** Experiment with different Ujjayi modifications as your belly grows. Try seated Ujjayi with hands supporting your belly, or modify it while standing or on all fours.

- **Visualization Breath:** Breathe deeply and imagine your breath flowing through your body, relaxing each muscle and preparing you for birth. Combine this with calming visualizations for added benefit.

Labor Stages:

- **Early Labor:** Ujjayi breath remains your go-to for managing mild contractions. Combine it with gentle movement or relaxation poses like Child's Pose.
- **Active Labor:** Maintain Ujjayi breath with deeper inhales and longer exhales as contractions intensify. Visualize your breath softening and opening your cervix.
- **Transition:** Short, rapid breaths like Kapalbhati can help manage intense contractions and provide quick bursts of energy.
- **Pushing:** Coordinate your Ujjayi breath with each push, using strong exhales to

power your efforts. Visualize your breath pushing your baby down and out.

- **Delivery:** Continue Ujjayi breath as needed, focusing on slow, deep breaths during birthing and recovery.

Remember:

- Listen to your body and modify techniques as needed. There's no "right" way to breathe – find what works for you.
- Practice regularly throughout your pregnancy to build familiarity and confidence with these techniques.
- Combine pranayama with mindfulness exercises for added benefit.

Embrace the power of your breath, mama! These pranayama techniques are your tools for navigating pregnancy and birth with awareness, strength, and peace. Remember, you are powerful, capable, and ready to birth your baby with grace and confidence. Breathe deeply, trust your body, and enjoy the incredible journey ahead!

any new breathing techniques, especially during pregnancy.

Chapter 12

Downward-Facing Diapers: Recovering Gracefully with Postpartum Yoga (Because #NewMomLife is Real)

Congratulations, mama! You've brought a beautiful miracle into the world, and now you're navigating the wonderful (and sometimes overwhelming) world of postpartum life. Sleep deprivation, endless diaper changes, and a body that feels like it's been through a warzone – it's enough to make even the most zen mama want to hide under the covers (with a giant mug of coffee). But fear not, warrior mama! Postpartum yoga is here to help you recover gracefully, reconnect with your body, and rediscover your inner strength – diaper duty and all.

Why Postpartum Yoga is Your Postpartum BFF:

- **Healing from the Inside Out:** Gentle yoga poses help strengthen your core muscles, improve pelvic floor function, and ease postpartum discomforts. Think of it as internal physiotherapy, helping your body heal and rebuild from the inside out.
- **Bonding with Your Body (and Your Baby!):** Postpartum yoga isn't just about physical recovery; it's about reconnecting with your body and appreciating its incredible journey. Bring your baby along for some skin-to-skin snuggles during supported poses, creating beautiful bonding moments.
- **Stress Slayer for Super Mamas:** Let's face it, new motherhood is stressful. Postpartum yoga incorporates mindfulness and relaxation techniques to combat stress, anxiety, and even baby blues. Imagine yourself inhaling peace and exhaling overwhelm – one exhale at a time.
- **Building a Support System:** Group postpartum yoga classes can connect you

with other mamas on the same journey. Share experiences, offer encouragement, and build a supportive community that understands the joys and challenges of new motherhood.

Postpartum Poses for New Mamas:

- **Supported Child's Pose:** A comforting and restorative pose that eases lower back pain and promotes relaxation. Use bolsters or pillows for extra support.
- **Cat-Cow:** This gentle spine mobilization improves flexibility and relieves tension. Bonus: it's a fun game for baby to watch!
- **Seated Twists:** Gentle twists stimulate digestion, improve circulation, and release tension in the back and shoulders. Modify with supported positions if needed.
- **Reclined Leg Raises:** Strengthen your core and pelvic floor muscles while lying comfortably on your back with legs extended. Start with small lifts and gradually increase as you feel stronger.

- **Supported Bridge Pose:** Opens your chest, strengthens your glutes and hamstrings, and improves circulation. Use bolsters or pillows for support under your hips and lower back.

Remember:

- **Listen to Your Body:** You're not the same mama you were pre-baby. Modify poses, take breaks, and prioritize your comfort above all else.
- **Clearance from Your Doc is Key:** Always consult your healthcare provider before starting any exercise program, especially after childbirth.
- **Be Patient and Kind:** Recovery takes time. Celebrate small victories, don't compare yourself to others, and focus on nurturing your body and mind with gentle kindness.
- **It's Not Just About Yoga:** Postpartum yoga is a wonderful tool, but it's not a magic bullet. Surround yourself with supportive loved ones, seek help when

needed, and remember, you're doing an amazing job, mama!

So, embrace the "downward-facing diaper" moments, mama. Postpartum yoga is your ally on this incredible journey of healing, self-discovery, and rediscovering your inner strength. Remember, you are powerful, capable, and worthy of love and care. Now go forth and conquer motherhood, one mindful breath and gentle pose at a time!

Disclaimer: Always consult your healthcare provider before starting any new exercise program, especially postpartum.

Chapter 13

Rebuilding Your Core: Gentle Strength Training for New Mamas (Because Your Core is More Than Just Abs)

Welcome back, mamas! You've embarked on the beautiful journey of motherhood, and while snuggles and endless love are definitely included, so are some physical changes. Your core muscles, which played a crucial role in pregnancy and childbirth, now need some TLC to heal and regain their strength. But fear not, mama! This chapter dives into gentle strength training exercises designed to rebuild your core without unnecessary strain or stress.

Beyond the Six-Pack: Redefining Core Strength:

Forget the picture-perfect six-pack often associated with "core strength." Your core is like a symphony orchestra, with numerous muscles working together to support your spine, pelvis, and overall stability. Postpartum core training focuses on **reactivating and strengthening these deeper muscles**, promoting healing, improving posture, and preventing future pain.

Why Gentle Strength Training is Key:

- **Healing from the Inside Out:** Gentle exercises stimulate blood flow, improve circulation, and promote healing of your abdominal muscles and pelvic floor. Think of it as physiotherapy for your core, strengthening from the inside out.

- **Preventing Future Woes:** A strong core reduces the risk of back pain, diastasis recti (separation of abdominal muscles), and pelvic floor dysfunction, setting you up for a healthier future. Imagine laying a strong foundation for your physical well-being.

- **Boosting Confidence & Energy:** Feeling strong and in control of your body can do wonders for your confidence and energy levels. Witness the power of feeling empowered and ready to tackle motherhood's challenges.

- **Building a Functional Core:** Forget crunches that strain your neck. We're focused on functional exercises that mimic everyday movements like lifting your baby or bending down to pick up toys. Imagine building a core that supports your daily life seamlessly.

Gentle Exercises for Postpartum Strength:

- **Bird-Dog:** Start on all fours, extend one arm and opposite leg simultaneously, keeping your core engaged and back flat. Repeat on the other side. This activates various core muscles without straining your back.
- **Plank Variations:** Begin with a modified plank on your forearms and knees. Gradually progress to a high plank on your toes as your strength improves. Plank variations strengthen your entire core without putting pressure on your abdominal muscles.

- **Pelvic Tilts:** Lie on your back with knees bent and feet flat on the floor. Gently tilt your pelvis up and down, engaging your core with each movement. This targets your pelvic floor muscles for improved function.
- **Side Plank:** Prop yourself up on one forearm with your body in a straight line from head to heels. Engage your core and hold for a few breaths. Repeat on the other side. This strengthens your obliques and improves overall core stability.
- **Walking Lunges:** Step forward with one leg, lowering your hips until both knees are bent at 90 degrees. Engage your core and push back to starting position. Repeat on the other side. This exercise works your core, glutes, and legs for functional strength.

Remember:

- **Listen to Your Body:** Start slowly and gradually increase intensity and duration as you feel stronger. Discomfort is a sign to modify or stop.

- **Clearance from Your Doc is Key:** Always consult your healthcare provider before starting any exercise program, especially postpartum.
- **Focus on Quality, Not Quantity:** It's not about how many reps you do, but about engaging your core with proper form. Quality movement over quantity!
- **Be Patient and Kind:** Rebuilding your core takes time. Celebrate small victories, don't compare yourself to others, and focus on gentle progress with self-compassion.

Remember, mama, your core is a masterpiece, intricately woven to support your body and motherhood journey. Embrace gentle strength training as a way to reconnect with your core, heal from within, and build a foundation for a strong and empowered future. You've got this, mama! Now go forth and conquer motherhood, one gentle exercise at a time.

any new exercise program, especially postpartum.

Chapter 14

Mama & Mini Flow: Bonding with Baby Through Yoga Practices (Because Cuddles & Playtime Can Be Yoga Too!)

Congratulations, super mama! You're navigating the incredible journey of motherhood, and now it's time to include your little bundle of joy in your yoga practice. This chapter explores the heartwarming world of "Mama & Mini Yoga," offering playful flows and bonding exercises that nurture the connection between you and your baby while promoting both your physical and emotional well-being.

Why Mama & Mini Yoga is Magical:

- **Building Stronger Bonds:** Sharing yoga moments with your baby strengthens the emotional connection, fostering trust, love, and joyful interactions. Imagine creating happy memories while nurturing your bond through movement and play.

- **Stimulating Baby's Development:** Gentle stretches and movements support your baby's physical development, improving motor skills, flexibility, and coordination. Think of it as playful physiotherapy for your little one!

- **Promoting Relaxation for Both:** Yoga postures and calming breaths can soothe both you and your baby, reducing stress and creating a peaceful space for connection. Picture yourselves melting into relaxation, one cuddle at a time.

- **Mommy Time (with a Twist):** Mama & Mini Yoga offers a unique opportunity to move your body, have fun with your baby, and enjoy some quality "me-time" that nurtures both of you. Imagine a workout that feels like playtime, filled with smiles and giggles.

Fun Flows for Tiny Yogis and Super Mamas:

- **Sunshine Stretch:** Lie on your back with baby on your chest. Gently lift your legs up and down, mimicking sunshine rays. Laugh and sing as you "warm" your baby with sunshine love.

- **Airplane Ride:** Hold baby securely on your forearm, "fly" around the room, making airplane noises and encouraging giggles. This playful movement strengthens your arms and engages baby's core.

- **Seated Cat-Cow:** Sit on the floor with baby on your lap. Move your spine up and down like a cat and cow, making animal sounds and encouraging baby to reach for your moving hands. This promotes spinal mobility and playful interaction.

- **Happy Baby Pose:** Lay baby on their back, hold their legs near their ankles, and gently rock them side to side. Sing soothing songs and watch their happy smiles emerge. This releases gas and promotes relaxation.

- **Supported Savasana:** Lie down on your back with baby snuggled next to you. Use blankets and pillows for support. Close your eyes, breathe deeply, and enjoy this peaceful cuddle moment. This promotes relaxation and bonding for both of you.

Remember:

- **Follow Your Baby's Lead:** Pay attention to your baby's cues and modify poses as needed. Stop if they seem uncomfortable or fussy.
- **Safety First:** Ensure a safe and comfortable environment with soft surfaces and plenty of space.
- **It's About Play, Not Perfection:** Don't worry about achieving perfect poses. Focus on fun, connection, and enjoying the moment with your little one.
- **Be Patient and Have Fun:** Enjoy the laughter, giggles, and occasional chaos that comes with Mama & Mini Yoga. These precious moments create lasting

memories and strengthen your bond in a unique and joyful way.

So, mama, embrace the magic of Mama & Mini Yoga! It's not just about poses, it's about creating heart-warming connections, playful movement, and shared moments of relaxation with your precious little one. Remember, you are both unique yogis on this incredible journey, and every smile, giggle, and cuddle is a perfect pose in itself. Now go forth and bond with your baby, one playful flow at a time!

Chapter 15

You Did It, Mama! Celebrating Your Journey and Looking Ahead

Congratulations, mama! You've reached the final chapter of this empowering journey we've shared. From navigating the whirlwind of pregnancy to embracing the joys and challenges of postpartum life, you've accomplished something truly remarkable. Take a moment to breathe deeply, acknowledge your strength, and celebrate the incredible transformation you've undergone.

Reflecting on Your Journey:

- **Celebrate Your Victories:** Remember every milestone, big or small. From mastering Ujjayi breath to soothing your fussy baby, acknowledge your triumphs and the incredible resilience you've shown.

- **Embrace the Challenges:** We all face bumps in the road. Reflect on the difficulties you overcame with grace and kindness, learning valuable lessons along the way.
- **Cherish the Memories:** Hold onto the moments that made your heart melt – your baby's first smile, the first cuddle, the laughter shared during Mama & Mini Yoga. These precious memories will forever nourish your soul.

Looking Ahead with Confidence:

- **Continue Your Yoga Journey:** Yoga is a lifelong practice. Find ways to incorporate movement and mindfulness into your routine, nurturing your well-being and connecting with your ever-evolving self.
- **Embrace the Village:** You are not alone. Build a supportive network of loved ones, fellow mamas, or online communities to share your joys, challenges, and unwavering strength.

- **Be Kind to Yourself:** Motherhood is a constant learning curve. Forgive yourself for mistakes, celebrate small wins, and shower yourself with the same love and compassion you give your child.

Remember, mama, you are:

- **Strong:** You've birthed a miracle and continue to nurture it with love and dedication.
- **Resilient:** You've faced challenges head-on and emerged stronger and wiser.
- **Empowered:** You have the knowledge and tools to navigate motherhood with confidence and grace.
- **Loved:** You are surrounded by love, from your precious child to your support system and yourself.

As you close this chapter and embark on new adventures, carry these affirmations in your heart. You are incredible, mama, and the world is a brighter place because of you. Go forth and

shine your light, one mindful breath and loving
embrace at a time.

Glossary of Yoga Terms for the Clueless Mama

Namaste, mama! This glossary is your handy guide to understanding some common yoga terms you might encounter on your postpartum journey. Remember, there's no need to feel overwhelmed – focus on enjoying the practice and connecting with your body and baby.

Asanas: The physical postures in yoga. Think of them as playful movements, not perfect poses.

Breathwork: Techniques like Ujjayi (oceanic breath) and Kapalbhati (breath of fire) that help regulate your nervous system and enhance your practice.

Cuddles & Playtime: Essential "poses" in Mama & Mini Yoga that strengthen your bond with your baby through movement and laughter.

Diaphragmatic Breathing: Deep breaths using your belly, not your chest, which promotes relaxation and oxygen flow.

Downward-Facing Dog: A fundamental pose where you start on all fours, lift your hips up, and create an inverted V shape. Modify with blocks or kneeling variations as needed.

Modifications: Anpassungen! Adjust any pose to fit your body and comfort level, especially postpartum. Don't be afraid to use props like bolsters, blankets, and blocks.

Namaste: A greeting and expression of respect, meaning "the divine in me bows to the divine in you." Feel free to namaste your baby, your reflection, or the world around you!

Om: A sacred sound chanted in yoga, often used to begin and end a practice. It's not about perfect pronunciation, but about the intention and feeling behind it.

Pranayama: Breathing exercises that control your breath for various benefits, like calming the mind or energizing the body. Think of it as mindful breathing with fancy names.

Relaxation Poses: Savasana (Corpse Pose) and Child's Pose are prime examples, encouraging deep rest and restoration. Snuggle your baby close and melt into relaxation together.

Savasana: The ultimate relaxation pose, lying flat on your back with arms at your sides. Think of it as a mini-vacation after a playful Mama & Mini flow.

Shavasana: Another name for Savasana, just like "namaste" and "the divine in me bows to the divine in you" mean the same thing. Yoga loves synonyms!

Supported Poses: Using bolsters, blankets, and blocks to prop up your body and make poses more comfortable and accessible, especially postpartum. Think of them as your supportive yoga friends.

Twists: Gentle spinal rotations that release tension and improve flexibility. Modify with supported variations to avoid straining your postpartum body.

Ujjayi Breath: The "oceanic breath" sound you make by constricting the back of your throat during exhales. It might feel weird at first, but practice makes progress!

Warrior Poses: Standing postures that build strength and stability. Think of them as empowering poses for the warrior mama you are!

Yogi/Yogini: Anyone who practices yoga, regardless of skill level. You are both yogis now, mama and mini!

Remember, mama, this is your yoga journey. Explore, have fun, and most importantly, be kind to yourself. You've got this!

Appendix

Sample Yoga Routines for Each Trimester

Disclaimer: It's important to consult with your healthcare provider before starting any new exercise program, especially during pregnancy. These routines are for informational purposes only and should be adapted to your individual needs and abilities.

First Trimester:

Focus: Gentle movement, stress reduction, and maintaining strength and flexibility.

Warm-up: 5-10 minutes of gentle stretches and walking in place.

Sun Salutations: Modified versions focusing on upper body movement and avoiding deep lunges.

Standing Poses: Warrior I & II with wide stances, Triangle Pose with modifications, Mountain Pose with gentle side bends.

Seated Poses: Seated Cat-Cow, Easy Pose with forward folds, Supported Child's Pose.

Floor Poses: Supported Bridge Pose, Side-lying Leg Lifts, Modified Downward-Facing Dog on forearms.

Cool-down: 5-10 minutes of deep breathing and Savasana (Corpse Pose) with modifications.

Second Trimester:

Focus: Maintaining flexibility, strengthening core and pelvic floor, and preparing for birth.

Warm-up: 5-10 minutes of dynamic stretches and walking lunges.

Sun Salutations: Full variations with modifications as needed (avoid jumping and deep lunges).

Standing Poses: Warrior I & II with wider stances, Triangle Pose with support, Tree Pose for balance.

Seated Poses: Seated Cat-Cow, Hero's Pose (Virasana) with modifications, Seated Twist poses with gentle rotations.

Floor Poses: Bridge Pose with variations, Cat-Cow on all fours, Modified Downward-Facing Dog on forearms or hands.

Cool-down: 5-10 minutes of deep breathing and supported Savasana.

Third Trimester:

Focus: Maintaining mobility, preparing for birth, and relaxation.

Warm-up: 5-10 minutes of gentle stretches and walking in place.

Modified Sun Salutations: Focus on upper body movements and avoid deep lunges.

Standing Poses: Wide-legged stances for Warrior I & II, supported Tree Pose, gentle side bends.

Seated Poses: Supported Seated Cat-Cow, Butterfly Pose (Baddha Konasana) with modifications, Supported Wide-Legged Forward Fold.

Floor Poses: Modified Plank on forearms, Cat-Cow on all fours, Child's Pose with variations, Supported Savasana.

Cool-down: 5-10 minutes of deep breathing and Savasana with plenty of pillows and bolsters for support.

Postpartum:

Focus: Gentle strengthening, rebuilding core and pelvic floor, and reconnecting with your body.

Warm-up: 5-10 minutes of gentle stretches and walking in place.

Pelvic Floor Exercises: Kegels and pelvic tilts focusing on activation and control.

Gentle Core Exercises: Bird-Dog pose, modified plank variations on forearms or knees.

Stretches: Cat-Cow on all fours, Child's Pose, supported hamstring stretches.

Seated Poses: Easy Pose with supported forward folds, Seated Twists with gentle rotations.

Floor Poses: Bridge Pose with modifications, Modified Downward-Facing Dog on forearms or hands.

Cool-down: 5-10 minutes of deep breathing and Savasana with modifications.

Remember: These are just examples, and you should adjust them based on your needs and capabilities. Listen to your body and take breaks whenever needed. Enjoy your practice!

Bonus

https://screenpal.com/watch/cZnI1FVdBbw
Video link for tutorials